KIDNEY DISEASE DIET COOKBOOK FOR SENIORS 2024

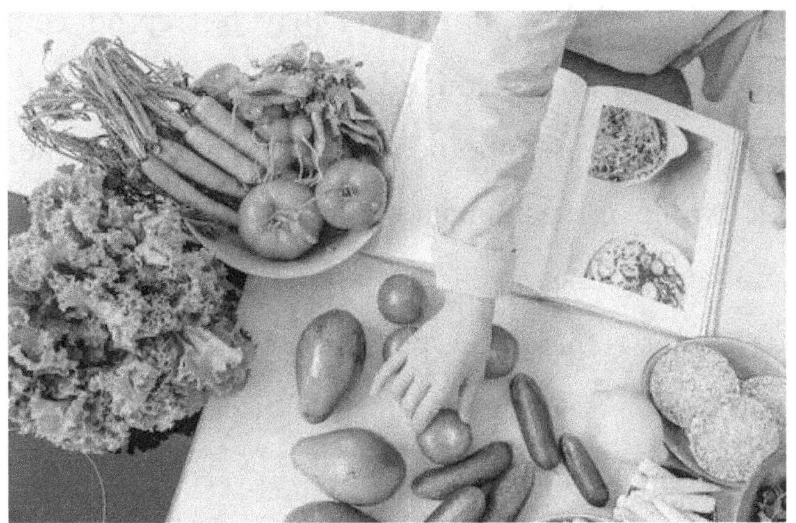

Healthy and Delicious Low Sodium, Potassium, and Phosphorus Recipes with Expert Tips for Managing Chronic Kidney Disease

Wilbert M. Jensen

GAIN ACCESS TO MORE BOOKS FROM ME

TABLE OF CONTENT

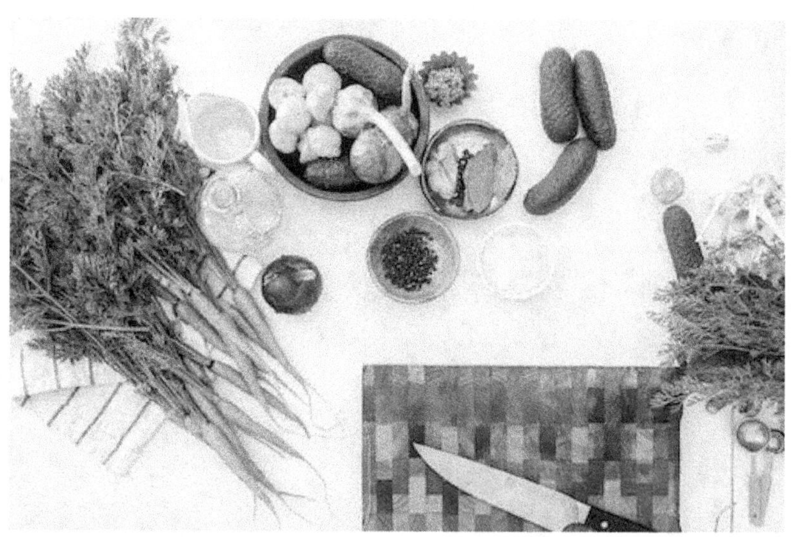

INTRODUCTION

Zoe, a retired nurse, had a new difficulty in her senior years: renal illness. Determined to keep her health and vigor, she began studying strategies to manage her disease. Zoe's expertise in healthcare helped her understand the significance of food in renal disease treatment.

She stumbled onto a renal illness diet cookbook designed for elders like herself. It became her go-to resource for creating tasty and kidney-friendly meals, along with nutritional recipes and useful recommendations.

Zoe enjoyed the cookbook, trying out delectable foods that matched her dietary limitations while also satisfying her taste buds.

Zoe's adventure with the cookbook not only restored her health, but also revealed a love of cooking. She shared her newfound knowledge with others in her senior community, encouraging them to take charge of their health by eating mindfully.

With each meal she cooked, Zoe demonstrated that with the correct resources and commitment, anybody can flourish despite medical problems.

DELICIOUS RECIPES KIDNEY DISEASE DIET COOKBOOK FOR SENIORS

Chicken and Vegetable Stir-Fry

Ingredients:

1 boneless, skinless chicken breast, thinly sliced

1 cup mixed vegetables (bell peppers, broccoli, carrots)

1 tablespoon olive oil

2 cloves garlic, minced

2 tablespoons low-sodium soy sauce

1 teaspoon ginger, grated

Salt and pepper to taste

Preparation:

Heat olive oil in a skillet over medium heat.

Add minced garlic and ginger, sauté until fragrant.

Add chicken slices, cook until browned.

Stir in mixed vegetables, cook until tender.

Pour in soy sauce, season with salt and pepper.

Cook for an additional 2-3 minutes, then serve.

Salmon with Lemon-Dill Sauce

Ingredients:

1 salmon fillet

1 tablespoon fresh dill, chopped

1 lemon, sliced

Salt and pepper to taste

Preparation:

Preheat oven to 375°F (190°C).

Place salmon fillet on a baking sheet lined with parchment paper.

Season with salt, pepper, and chopped dill.

Top with lemon slices.

Bake for 15-20 minutes or until salmon is cooked through.

Serve hot with additional lemon slices if desired.

Quinoa and Black Bean Salad

Ingredients:

1 cup quinoa, rinsed

1 can black beans, drained and rinsed

1 red bell pepper, diced

1/4 cup red onion, finely chopped

1/4 cup fresh cilantro, chopped

2 tablespoons olive oil

2 tablespoons lime juice

Salt and pepper to taste

Preparation:

Cook quinoa according to package instructions, let it cool.

In a large bowl, combine cooked quinoa, black beans, diced bell pepper, chopped red onion, and cilantro.

In a small bowl, whisk together olive oil, lime juice, salt, and pepper.

Pour the dressing over the salad and toss to combine.

Serve chilled or at room temperature.

Turkey and Vegetable Soup

Ingredients:

1 pound ground turkey

1 onion, diced

2 carrots, sliced

2 celery stalks, sliced

4 cups low-sodium chicken broth

1 can diced tomatoes

1 teaspoon dried thyme

Salt and pepper to taste

Preparation:

In a large pot, brown ground turkey over medium heat.

Add diced onion, sliced carrots, and celery, cook until vegetables are tender.

Pour in chicken broth and diced tomatoes, bring to a simmer.

Stir in dried thyme, salt, and pepper.

Let the soup simmer for 20-30 minutes.

Serve hot and enjoy.

Eggplant Parmesan

Ingredients:

1 large eggplant, sliced into rounds

1 cup whole wheat breadcrumbs

1/2 cup grated Parmesan cheese

2 eggs, beaten

2 cups marinara sauce

1 cup shredded mozzarella cheese

Fresh basil leaves for garnish

Preparation:

Preheat oven to 375°F (190°C).

Dip eggplant slices in beaten eggs, then coat with breadcrumbs mixed with Parmesan cheese.

Place coated eggplant slices on a baking sheet lined with parchment paper.

Bake for 20-25 minutes or until golden brown and crispy.

In a baking dish, spread a layer of marinara sauce.

Arrange baked eggplant slices on top of the sauce, then top with remaining marinara sauce and shredded mozzarella cheese.

Bake for an additional 15-20 minutes until cheese is melted and bubbly.

Garnish with fresh basil leaves before serving.

Spinach and Feta Stuffed Chicken Breast

Ingredients:

2 boneless, skinless chicken breasts

2 cups fresh spinach leaves

1/4 cup crumbled feta cheese

1 clove garlic, minced

1 tablespoon olive oil

Salt and pepper to taste

Preparation:

Preheat oven to 375°F (190°C).

Make a pocket in each chicken breast by slicing horizontally.

In a skillet, heat olive oil over medium heat.

Add minced garlic and spinach leaves, cook until wilted.

Remove from heat and let cool slightly.

Stuff each chicken breast with cooked spinach and crumbled feta cheese.

Season the outside of the chicken breasts with salt and pepper.

Place stuffed chicken breasts on a baking sheet lined with parchment paper.

Bake for 25-30 minutes or until chicken is cooked through.

Serve hot with your favorite side dishes.

Vegetable and Bean Chili

Ingredients:

1 tablespoon olive oil

1 onion, diced

2 cloves garlic, minced

1 bell pepper, diced

1 zucchini, diced

1 can kidney beans, drained and rinsed

1 can black beans, drained and rinsed

1 can diced tomatoes

2 tablespoons chili powder

1 teaspoon cumin

Salt and pepper to taste

Preparation:

Heat olive oil in a large pot over medium heat.

Add diced onion and minced garlic, sauté until fragrant.

Stir in diced bell pepper and zucchini, cook until softened.

Add drained and rinsed kidney beans, black beans, and diced tomatoes to the pot.

Season with chili powder, cumin, salt, and pepper.

Let the chili simmer for 20-30 minutes, stirring occasionally.

Serve hot with your favorite toppings such as shredded cheese, sour cream, or fresh cilantro.

Lemon Herb Grilled Chicken

Ingredients:

2 boneless, skinless chicken breasts

Juice of 1 lemon

2 tablespoons olive oil

2 cloves garlic, minced

1 teaspoon dried thyme

1 teaspoon dried rosemary

Salt and pepper to taste

Preparation:

In a small bowl, whisk together lemon juice, olive oil, minced garlic, dried thyme, dried rosemary, salt, and pepper.

Place chicken breasts in a shallow dish and pour the marinade over them.

Cover and refrigerate for at least 30 minutes, or up to 4 hours.

Preheat grill to medium-high heat.

Remove chicken from marinade and discard excess marinade.

Grill chicken for 6-7 minutes per side, or until cooked through and no longer pink in the center.

Let chicken rest for a few minutes before serving.

Slice and serve with your favorite side dishes.

Mediterranean Chickpea Salad

Ingredients:

1 can chickpeas, drained and rinsed

1 cucumber, diced

1 bell pepper, diced

1/4 cup red onion, finely chopped

1/4 cup Kalamata olives, sliced

1/4 cup crumbled feta cheese

2 tablespoons olive oil

2 tablespoons red wine vinegar

1 teaspoon dried oregano

Salt and pepper to taste

Preparation:

In a large bowl, combine chickpeas, diced cucumber, diced bell pepper, chopped red onion, sliced Kalamata olives, and crumbled feta cheese.

In a small bowl, whisk together olive oil, red wine vinegar, dried oregano, salt, and pepper.

Pour the dressing over the salad and toss to combine.

Serve chilled or at room temperature.

Turkey Meatballs with Marinara Sauce

Ingredients:

1 pound ground turkey

1/2 cup breadcrumbs

1/4 cup grated Parmesan cheese

1 egg, beaten

2 cloves garlic, minced

1 teaspoon dried oregano

1/2 teaspoon dried basil

Salt and pepper to taste

2 cups marinara sauce

Preparation:

Preheat oven to 375°F (190°C).

In a large bowl, combine ground turkey, breadcrumbs, grated Parmesan cheese, beaten egg, minced garlic, dried oregano, dried basil, salt, and pepper.

Mix until well combined, then shape the mixture into meatballs.

Place meatballs on a baking sheet lined with parchment paper.

Bake for 20-25 minutes or until cooked through.

Heat marinara sauce in a saucepan over medium heat.

Add cooked meatballs to the marinara sauce and simmer for 5-10 minutes.

Serve hot with your favorite pasta or vegetable side dish.

Sesame Ginger Tofu Stir-Fry

Ingredients:

1 block extra-firm tofu, cubed

1 cup mixed vegetables (snap peas, bell peppers, carrots)

2 tablespoons sesame oil

2 tablespoons low-sodium soy sauce

1 tablespoon honey

1 teaspoon fresh ginger, grated

2 cloves garlic, minced

1 tablespoon sesame seeds

Salt and pepper to taste

Preparation:

Press tofu to remove excess moisture, then cut into cubes.

Heat sesame oil in a skillet over medium heat.

Add minced garlic and grated ginger, sauté until fragrant.

Add cubed tofu to the skillet, cook until lightly browned on all sides.

Stir in mixed vegetables and cook until tender.

In a small bowl, whisk together soy sauce and honey.

Pour the sauce over the tofu and vegetables, toss to coat evenly.

Sprinkle sesame seeds over the stir-fry and season with salt and pepper.

Cook for an additional 2-3 minutes, then serve hot with rice or noodles.

Greek Salad with Grilled Chicken

Ingredients:

2 boneless, skinless chicken breasts

4 cups mixed greens (lettuce, spinach, arugula)

1 cucumber, sliced

1 tomato, diced

1/4 cup red onion, thinly sliced

1/4 cup Kalamata olives

1/4 cup crumbled feta cheese

2 tablespoons olive oil

2 tablespoons red wine vinegar

1 teaspoon dried oregano

Salt and pepper to taste

Preparation:

Preheat grill to medium-high heat.

Season chicken breasts with salt, pepper, and dried oregano.

Grill chicken for 6-7 minutes per side, or until cooked through.

Let chicken rest for a few minutes, then slice.

In a large bowl, combine mixed greens, sliced cucumber, diced tomato, thinly sliced red onion, Kalamata olives, and crumbled feta cheese.

In a small bowl, whisk together olive oil, red wine vinegar, dried oregano, salt, and pepper.

Pour the dressing over the salad and toss to combine.

Divide salad onto plates and top with grilled chicken slices.

Lentil and Vegetable Soup

Ingredients:

1 cup green lentils, rinsed

1 onion, diced

2 carrots, sliced

2 celery stalks, sliced

4 cups vegetable broth

1 can diced tomatoes

2 cloves garlic, minced

1 teaspoon dried thyme

1 teaspoon paprika

Salt and pepper to taste

Preparation:

In a large pot, heat olive oil over medium heat.

Add diced onion and minced garlic, sauté until fragrant.

Stir in sliced carrots and celery, cook until softened.

Add rinsed green lentils, vegetable broth, diced tomatoes, dried thyme, paprika, salt, and pepper to the pot.

Bring the soup to a boil, then reduce heat and let it simmer for 20-25 minutes, or until lentils are tender.

Adjust seasoning if needed, then serve hot.

Roasted Vegetable Quinoa Bowl

Ingredients:

1 cup quinoa, rinsed

2 cups mixed vegetables (zucchini, bell peppers, cherry tomatoes)

2 tablespoons olive oil

1 teaspoon dried thyme

Salt and pepper to taste

Preparation:

Preheat oven to 400°F (200°C).

Place mixed vegetables on a baking sheet lined with parchment paper.

Drizzle olive oil over the vegetables and sprinkle with dried thyme, salt, and pepper.

Toss to coat evenly, then spread the vegetables in a single layer.

Roast in the preheated oven for 20-25 minutes or until vegetables are tender and lightly browned.

Meanwhile, cook quinoa according to package instructions.

Once quinoa and vegetables are cooked, divide quinoa into bowls and top with roasted vegetables.

Serve hot as a nutritious and flavorful meal.

Turkey and Spinach Stuffed Bell Peppers

Ingredients:

4 bell peppers (any color), halved and seeded

1 pound ground turkey

1 onion, diced

2 cloves garlic, minced

2 cups fresh spinach leaves, chopped

1 can diced tomatoes

1 cup cooked quinoa

1 teaspoon dried Italian seasoning

Salt and pepper to taste

1/2 cup shredded mozzarella cheese

Preparation:

Preheat oven to 375°F (190°C).

In a skillet, brown ground turkey over medium heat.

Add diced onion and minced garlic, cook until softened.

Stir in chopped spinach leaves and diced tomatoes, cook until spinach is wilted.

Remove from heat and stir in cooked quinoa, dried Italian seasoning, salt, and pepper.

Spoon turkey and spinach mixture into halved bell peppers.

Place stuffed bell peppers in a baking dish, then sprinkle shredded mozzarella cheese on top.

Cover the baking dish with aluminum foil and bake for 25-30 minutes.

Remove foil and bake for an additional 5-10 minutes or until cheese is melted and bubbly.

Serve hot as a satisfying and nutritious meal.

Vegetable Fried Rice

Ingredients:

2 cups cooked brown rice

1 cup mixed vegetables (peas, carrots, corn)

2 eggs, beaten

2 tablespoons low-sodium soy sauce

1 tablespoon sesame oil

2 cloves garlic, minced

2 green onions, thinly sliced

Salt and pepper to taste

Preparation:

Heat sesame oil in a large skillet or wok over medium heat.

Add minced garlic and sliced green onions, sauté until fragrant.

Push garlic and green onions to one side of the skillet, then pour beaten eggs into the empty side.

Scramble eggs until cooked through, then mix with garlic and green onions.

Add mixed vegetables to the skillet and stir-fry until tender.

Stir in cooked brown rice and soy sauce, toss to combine.

Season with salt and pepper to taste.

Cook for an additional 2-3 minutes, then serve hot as a delicious and nutritious meal.

Baked Cod with Herbed Crust

Ingredients:

4 cod fillets

1/2 cup breadcrumbs

2 tablespoons grated Parmesan cheese

1 teaspoon dried parsley

1 teaspoon dried dill

1 teaspoon dried thyme

2 tablespoons olive oil

Salt and pepper to taste

Lemon wedges for serving

Preparation:

Preheat oven to 400°F (200°C).

In a bowl, combine breadcrumbs, grated Parmesan cheese, dried parsley, dried dill, dried thyme, salt, and pepper.

Pat cod fillets dry with paper towels, then brush with olive oil.

Press the breadcrumb mixture onto the top of each cod fillet to form a crust.

Place cod fillets on a baking sheet lined with parchment paper.

Bake for 12-15 minutes or until fish is cooked through and flakes easily with a fork.

Serve hot with lemon wedges for squeezing over the top.

Vegetable and Tofu Stir-Fry

Ingredients:

1 block extra-firm tofu, cubed

2 cups mixed vegetables (broccoli, bell peppers, snow peas)

2 tablespoons low-sodium soy sauce

1 tablespoon hoisin sauce

1 tablespoon sesame oil

2 cloves garlic, minced

1 teaspoon fresh ginger, grated

Salt and pepper to taste

Preparation:

Press tofu to remove excess moisture, then cut into cubes.

Heat sesame oil in a skillet or wok over medium heat.

Add minced garlic and grated ginger, sauté until fragrant.

Add cubed tofu to the skillet and cook until lightly browned on all sides.

Stir in mixed vegetables and cook until tender-crisp.

In a small bowl, whisk together soy sauce and hoisin sauce.

Pour the sauce over the tofu and vegetables, toss to coat evenly.

Season with salt and pepper to taste.

Cook for an additional 2-3 minutes, then serve hot with rice or noodles.

Tomato Basil Mozzarella Salad

Ingredients:

2 large tomatoes, sliced

1 ball fresh mozzarella cheese, sliced

1/4 cup fresh basil leaves

2 tablespoons balsamic glaze

Salt and pepper to taste

Preparation:

Arrange tomato slices and mozzarella slices alternately on a serving platter.

Tuck fresh basil leaves between the tomato and mozzarella slices.

Drizzle balsamic glaze over the salad.

Season with salt and pepper to taste.

Serve immediately as a refreshing and flavorful appetizer or side dish.

Sweet Potato and Black Bean Enchiladas

Ingredients:

2 large sweet potatoes, peeled and diced

1 can black beans, drained and rinsed

1 onion, diced

2 cloves garlic, minced

1 bell pepper, diced

1 cup enchilada sauce

8 whole wheat tortillas

1 cup shredded cheddar cheese

Fresh cilantro for garnish

Salt and pepper to taste

Preparation:

Preheat oven to 375°F (190°C).

Steam diced sweet potatoes until tender, then mash them in a bowl.

In a skillet, sauté diced onion, minced garlic, and diced bell pepper until softened.

Stir in black beans and mashed sweet potatoes, season with salt and pepper.

Spread a spoonful of enchilada sauce on the bottom of a baking dish.

Fill each whole wheat tortilla with the sweet potato and black bean mixture, then roll up and place seam-side down in the baking dish.

Pour remaining enchilada sauce over the rolled tortillas, then sprinkle shredded cheddar cheese on top.

Cover the baking dish with aluminum foil and bake for 20-25 minutes.

Remove foil and bake for an additional 5-10 minutes until cheese is melted and bubbly.

Garnish with fresh cilantro before serving.

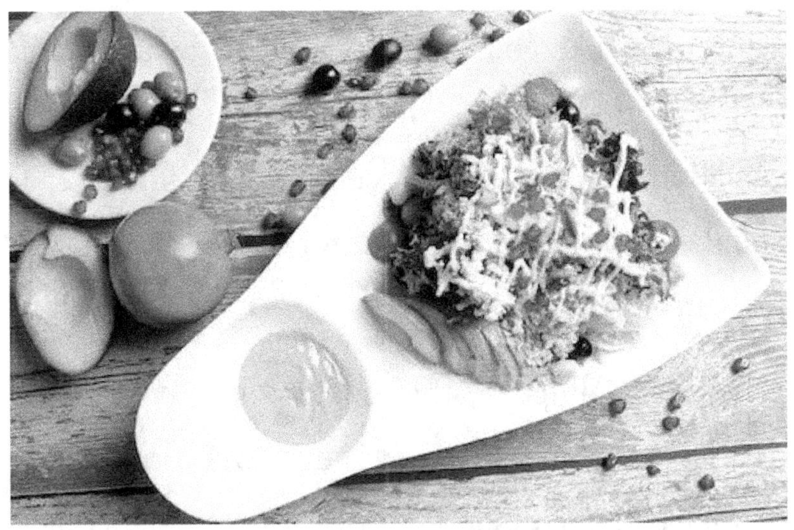

CONCLUSION

Nutrition is extremely important in the management of renal disease. This cookbook is more than just a collection of recipes; it is a source of hope and a road map to wellbeing for seniors dealing with renal health issues.

Each meal becomes a monument to tenacity and determination thanks to meticulous ingredient selection and attentive cooking techniques. It enables seniors to regain control of their health, one tasty meal at a time.

Beyond the kitchen, this cookbook encourages a feeling of community by connecting others on similar paths and sharing tales, achievements, and support. It serves as a reminder that, while kidney illness might create challenges, it does not define a person's path.

With devotion and the correct equipment, seniors may enjoy every minute, nurturing not just their bodies but also their spirits. This cookbook demonstrates the power of food, the strength of community, and the unfailing tenacity of the human spirit.

Happy cooking!

Contact me here